Manwar Al-Naqqash
Ahmed Al-Shewered
Rasha Al-Saad

Chemoradiation Roles in the Management of Rectal cancer

Manwar Al-Naqqash
Ahmed Al-Shewered
Rasha Al-Saad

Chemoradiation Roles in the Management of Rectal cancer

Systematic Review and Meta-analysis Study of Rectal cancer in Iraq

Noor Publishing

Imprint
Any brand names and product names mentioned in this book are subject to trademark, brand or patent protection and are trademarks or registered trademarks of their respective holders. The use of brand names, product names, common names, trade names, product descriptions etc. even without a particular marking in this work is in no way to be construed to mean that such names may be regarded as unrestricted in respect of trademark and brand protection legislation and could thus be used by anyone.

Cover image: www.ingimage.com

Publisher:
Noor Publishing
is a trademark of
International Book Market Service Ltd., member of OmniScriptum Publishing Group
17 Meldrum Street, Beau Bassin 71504, Mauritius
Printed at: see last page
ISBN: 978-620-0-77724-9

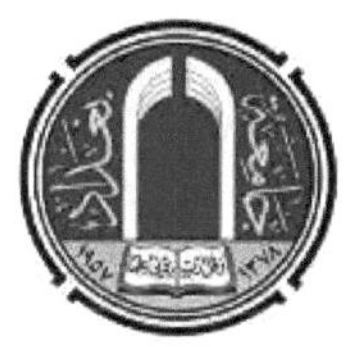

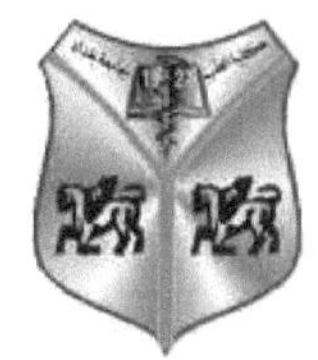

Ministry of Higher Education
and Scientific Research
University of Baghdad
College of Medicine

Chemoradiation Roles in the Management of Rectal cancer: Systematic Review and Meta-analysis Study in Medical City

Ahmed Salih Alshewered

Acknowledgements

It's from absolute oneness of God from no god but Allah alone. I thank God for his support and influence on my life and work. Not only, He did provide the project of my interest, and He encouraged me through the assistance of the expertise of many knowledgeable and caring people. I have blessed with the presence of many people who have assisted me with this research.

I would like to express my deep appreciation and sincere thanks to my supervisor's **Ass. Prof. Dr. Manwar Abdulelah Al-Naqqash** for helping and guiding me during the course of the work.

Sincere thanks are presented to my colleagues in post-graduate students and in the hostile for their support and assistance to finish my work.

Special thanks and regards for the ongoing support of my family, who did not spare the least effort to bring this work to light.

Detication

To

My Late Father

Beloved Mother

Lovely Wife

Five Little Angles

List of contents

List of tables

List of figures

List of abbreviations

5FU	Fluorouracil
APR	Abdominal perineal resection
CBC	Complete blood count
CRT	Chemoradiation
CT	Computed tomography
DFS	Disease free survival
ERUS	Endoscopic rectal ultrasound
FNA	Fine needle aspiration
IBD	Inflammatory bowel diseases
ICR	Iraqi Cancer Registry
LAR	Lower anterior resection
LFT	Liver function tests
MRI	Magnetic resonance imaging
N-O	Newcastle-Ottawa
OS	Overall survival
PRISMA	Preferred Reporting Items for Systematic Reviews and Meta-Analyses
r	Spearman correlation
RFT	Renal function tests
RT	Radiotherapy
TME	Total mesorectal excision
x^2	Chi-sequare

Abstract

Background: Rectal cancer is one of the most common malignant tumors of gastrointestinal tract. Chemoradiation (CRT) has a sound effect on its management.

Objectives: Assessment the patterns of characterizations of rectal cancer. Evaluation of the efficacy, and long-term survival of pre-/ postoperative CRT by collecting all eligible evidence articles and summarize the results.

Methods: By this systematic review and meta-analysis study, we include data of CRT of rectal cancer articles from 2015 until 2019. The research was carried out at Baghdad Medical City oncology centers. Accordance with the PRISMA guidelines, and the Newcastle-Ottawa Scale used.

Results: Starting with the gender distribution as M:F ratio of 0.94:1.06. Regarding the age, we recorded mean±SD of 48.7±14.2 years. Rectosigmoid represented the most common site as 50(49.5%), and adenocarcinoma was common histopathology as 76(75.2%) of patients, with localized stage in 50(49.5%). The moderate differentiation was most grade as 65(64.4%). The distant from anal verge mostly seen 5-10 cm in 59(58.4%). The pulmonary was commonest site of metastasis in 11(10.9%). Most patients undergo APR operation, which has done in 41(40.6%). Adjuvant CRT received by 40(39.6%) patients, whereas neoadjuvant CRT gave to 25 patients. A total of 2,609 articles from 12 databases met our search strategies. The highest Newcastle-Ottawa score (8) demonstrated in three studies, and median score (7) calculated in five studies.

Conclusions: The incidence belonged to 5th and 6th decade of life. Rectosigmoid represented the most common site. Mostly, the 5-10 cm distant of tumor from anal verge was common. The pulmonary was most site of metastasis. We concluded the formulation of a novel point that survival benefit found in many pre or postoperative CRT trials in rectal cancer with preform more for neoadjuvant sitting.

Keywords: **Rectal cancer, Chemoradiation, Rectosigmoid, TME, APR**

Introduction and Review of Literature

1.2. Rectal carcinoma

1.2.1. Anatomy

The rectum is about 15-16 cm long, and is subdivided into three parts according to the distance from the anal verge: upper third, from 12th to 16th cm; middle third, from 6th to 12th cm, and lower third, from 1st to 6th cm [1]. The anorectal ring (dentate line) is located at the level of the puborectalis sling and levators, representing the pelvic floor from within the pelvis [1]. The layer of mesorectal fascia encloses both the rectum and mesorectum with the perirectal lymph nodes [1].

1.2.2. Epidemiology

In 2011 recorded 1086 cases of colorectal cancer by the Iraqi Cancer Registry (ICR), as 5.3% of most ten cancer types in Iraq, whereas in 2015 the ICR recorded 1454 patients as 5.7% [2, 3]. Globally the new cases are diagnosed at 2018 worldwide, accounting 704,376 (3.9%) of human cancers [4]. Peak incidence rates are observed in Europe, while lowest incidence rates were noted in India, and South America and among Arab citizens. The risk increase with age, but 3-5 % can occur in patients younger than 40 years of age [1].

1.2.3. Etiology [1, 5, 6]

1. Polyps: Most rectal cancers arise from benign adenomatous polyps.
2. Diet: High intake of fat, higher caloric intakes, and low intake of fiber.
3. Environmental factors: migrant populations, from low-incidence regions in Africa and Asia to the high-incidence regions of North America.
4. Genetic factors: Family history recorded in 15% of all, associated with first-degree relatives.
5. Smoking: Twice to trice time increase the risk of cancer.

1.2.4. Histopathology

The majority (>90%) of colorectal cancers are adenocarcinomas. Some adenocarcinomas have mucin, which can be extracellular (colloid) or intracellular (signet-ring cell) [1, 6]. Colloid cancer, which occurs in 15-20%, whereas signet-ring cell carcinoma, which occurs in 1-2% [5]. Other histologic types are rare and include carcinoid tumors, leiomyosarcomas, lymphomas, and squamous cell cancers [5].

1.2.5. Clinical manifestations

The common symptoms include gross red blood (mixed or covering the stool, or by itself, sometimes accompanied by the passage of mucus) and a change in bowel habits such as unexplained constipation, diarrhea, or narrowing stool caliber [1, 6]. Hemorrhoidal bleeding should always be a diagnosis of exclusion [6]. Obstructing rectal cancers frequently present with diarrhea rather than constipation [6].

1.2.6. Diagnosis [1, 5, 6]

1. A comprehensive evaluation includes a complete physical examination with a digital rectal examination, CBC, LFT, and RFT.
2. Biopsy confirmation via colonoscopy or via CT-guided FNA.
3. CT or MRI with a contrast of the chest, abdomen, and pelvis.
4. Endoscopy for assessed the entire colonic mucosa because some patients have synchronous colorectal cancers and a more significant, have additional premalignant conditions.
5. ERUS significantly improves the preoperative assessment of the depth of invasion of large bowel tumors. The accuracy rate is 95% for ERUS, 70% for CT, and 60% for a digital rectal examination. The combination of ERUS to assess tumor extent and digital rectal exam to determine mobility should enable precise planning of surgical treatment and definition of those patients who may benefit from preoperative chemoradiation (T3, 4 and N+). Trans-rectal biopsy of perirectal lymph nodes can often be accomplished under EUS direction. MRI with rectal coils is comparable to ERUS in its sensitivity for staging the primary tumor and might be superior to ERUS in the identification of perirectal lymph node metastases.

1.2.7. Management

1.2.7.1. Surgery

The primary therapy for potentially curative rectal cancer is surgery [7]. Curative surgery should excise the tumor with wide margins and maximize regional lymphadenectomy such that at least 12-15 lymph nodes are available for pathologic evaluation [6]. Treatment options for rectal tumors include the following [6-10]:

1. Anterior resection of the rectum: Middle and upper rectum (6 to 15 cm).
2. Lower rectum (0 to 5 cm): Coloanal anastomosis, with or without a pouch, transanal excision, transsphincteric, and parasacral approaches, or abdominoperineal resection (APR).
3. Total mesorectal excision (TME): Data suggest that local recurrence rates may be decreased with *en bloc* sharp dissection of the entire mesorectum at the time of tumor destruction, and this procedure has now become standard. With this type of surgery, local control rates have markedly increased. However, even with TME, the local failure rate for the pathologic node-positive disease is 21%, and adjuvant chemoradiation is still necessary.

1.2.7.2. Neoadjuvant therapy

The current standard therapy for stage III rectal cancer, and sometimes for stage II disease, is preoperative chemotherapy using 5-FU and RT, followed by surgery, and then followed by adjuvant chemotherapy [11]. Because of the anatomic confines of the pelvic bones and sacrum, surgeons often cannot achieve wide, tumor-free margins during the resection of rectal cancer. Patients who have a complete pathologic response to preoperative therapy have a favorable long-term prognosis [6, 8-10].

1.2.7.3. Radiotherapy

As the primary and only treatment modality for small, mobile rectal tumors or in combination with chemotherapy after resection of rectal tumors. RT in palliative doses relieves pain, obstruction, bleeding, and tenesmus in about 80% of cases [6, 8-10].

1.2.7.4. Chemotherapy

The most commonly used chemotherapeutic agents are 5-FU (alone or in combination with leucovorin), capecitabine, irinotecan, and oxaliplatin [1, 5, 6, 8-10]. Regimens being used are:

1. 5-FU plus leucovorin.
2. CapeOX (oxaliplatine+capecitabine).
3. mFOLFOX6: Folinic acid (leucovorin), 5-FU, and oxaliplatin.
4. IFL: Irinotecan with 5-FU, and leucovorin.
5. FOLFIRI: Irinotecan, followed by folinic acid (leucovorin), and then 5-FU.
6. FOLFOX4: Folinic acid, 5-FU, and oxaliplatin.
7. IROX: Irinotecan + oxaliplatin.

For those with advanced stages, all regimens can be used, whereas in metastatic setting addition of Bevacizumab or Panitumumab or cetuximab can be of benefit [5]. The continuous IV infusion of 5-FU had been used to change the toxicity profile from hematologic to predominantly mucositis and dermatologic (hand–foot syndrome) when compared with bolus administration [5, 10]. The used irinotecan, which has been shown to improve survival and quality of life. In patients with recurrent disease refractory to at least one 5-FU regimen, the survival at one year of patients treated with supportive care alone or with 5-FU was about 15%, compared with 36% when patients were treated with irinotecan [5, 8-10].

1.2.7.5. Chemoradiation

Chemoradiation (RT+ 5FU or capecitabine) can be used preoperatively or postoperatively [1, 5]. For patients with the cT1-2N0 disease, the initial treatment is surgery, and if the tumor is pT3-4N0 or T any N1-2, this is commonly followed by postoperative chemoradiation [5, 9, 10]. For patients with cT3-4N0 or T any+ lesions, preoperative chemoradiation is given, followed by surgery and postoperative adjuvant chemotherapy [6, 10].

1.2.7.6. Chemoirradiation Trialists

GITSG 7175 deal with stage B2-C rectal CA randomized postoperatively to no adjuvant therapy vs. chemo alone vs. RT alone vs. concurrent chemoradiation. Chemoradiation arm improved 5-year DFS and OS over control [1, 5, 8-10].

The **National Cancer Institute (NCI) and Mayo/NCCTG 79-47-51** concluded in 1990 that chemoradiation was the standard postoperative adjuvant treatment for all patients with pT3 or N1-2 disease, and demonstrated improvements in both DFS and OS [5, 10, 11].

The **NSABP R-01, R-02** reported rectal cancer with B-C (II-III) treated with surgery alone vs. post-op RT vs. post-op chemo. RT improved LF (25 vs16%), while chemo improved DFS (30 vs 42%) and OS (43 vs 53%) vs. observation. Whereas **NSABP R-04** trial compared preoperative chemoradiation with 5-FU to capecitabine (with or without oxaliplatin), which had similar rates of pCR (22% versus 19%), sphincter sparing surgery (63% versus 61%), and grade 3 + diarrhea (11%) [5, 6, 8-10].

The **European Organization for Research and Treatment of Cancer (EORTC)** trial 22921 was a four-arm randomized trial found a significant decrease in the local failure rate in those patients who receive chemoradiation compared with irradiation (8% to 10% versus 17%; $p < 0.001$) but no difference in the 5-year OS (65%) [1, 5, 10, 12].

The **Fédération Francophone de la Cancérologie Digestive (FFCD 9203)** trial was a two-arm trial demonstrated the same decrease in local failure rates (8% versus 17%; $p < 0.05$) and a corresponding increase in pCR (11% versus 4%; $p < 0.05$) with preoperative compared to irradiation alone but no survival benefits (68% versus 67%) [5, 9, 10, 12].

The **NSABP R0-354** and the **German CAO/ ARO/AIO 94** trials were based on pilot data suggesting that chemotherapy increased the response rate of preoperative radiation, and because of less small bowel in the radiation field, the acute toxicity of preoperative chemoirradiation was less then postoperative chemoirradiation [5, 8-10, 14]. Patients who received preoperative therapy had a significant decrease in rates of local failure (6% versus 13%; $p = 0.006$), acute toxicity (27% versus 40%; $p = 0.001$), and chronic toxicity (14% versus 24%; $p = 0.012$).

The **STAR-01**, **ACCORD**, and **NSABP R-04** trials, when patient received oxaliplatin-based chemoirradiation had a significant improvement in pCR (17% versus 13%, $p = 0.045$) with no corresponding increase in acute grade 3+ toxicity (23% versus 22%) [8-10, 15, 16].

The **NSABP R-03** study accrued only those patients with cT3-4 rectal cancers [15, 16]. Patients who received preoperative versus postoperative therapy had a significant improvement in 5-year DFS (65% versus 53%; $p = 0.011$) and a borderline significant improvement in 5-year OS (75% versus 66%; $p = 0.065$).

The **UK Medical Research Council trial (MRC CR07)** randomized patients with clinical stages I to III rectal cancer to preoperative irradiation or selective postoperative chemoirradiation. With a median follow-up of 4 years, patients who received preoperative compared with selective postoperative treatment had significantly lower 3-year local recurrence rates (4.4% versus 10.6%; $p < 0.0001$) and higher 3-year DFS (77.5% versus 71.5%; $p = 0.013$) [15].

Short-course radiation (25 Gy in 5 fractions) was established as a standard therapy in the **Dutch Colorectal Cancer Group CKVO** and **Swedish Rectal Cancer** trials and chemoirradiation was created as a standard therapy by the **German Rectal Cancer Trial CAO/ARO/ AIO-94** (45-50.4 Gy in 25 to 28 fractions plus concurrent chemotherapy) [5, 10, 15, 16].

Polish Colorectal Study Group trial randomized patients with cT3 rectal cancers to preoperative short-course radiation compared to chemoirradiation [5, 8-10]. This showed a higher pCR rate (16% versus 1%) and a lower incidence of positive radial margins (4% versus 13%, $p = 0.017$). However, there were no significant differences in sphincter preservation (58% versus 61%), local recurrence (14% versus 9%), DFS (56% versus 58%) and 4-year OS (66% versus 67%) [11, 17].

Pooled-analysis on NCCTG trials, Int 0144, NSABP RO1, and RO2, revealed that post-op chemo appeared to improve OS, similar to post-op chemoradiation. DFS, OS, and LF tended to be better with chemoradiation [5, 8-10, 18].

1.3. Aims of the study

1. Assessment the patterns of distribution, characterizations, and management of rectal cancer.
2. Performing a comparing analysis between neoadjuvant and adjuvant chemoradiation in rectal cancer.
3. Collecting and analyzing all eligible evidence articles that fit for inclusion and exclusion criteria of Chemoradiation roles in rectal cancer.
4. Using a statistical methods and graphs to summarize the results of studies including.

Methods

2.1. Study setting

In this systematic review and meta-analysis study, the trials, and comparison studies that included data of chemoradiation roles in the management of rectal cancer were included, which were the results related to the subject of our research, with time limitations from 2015 until 2019. Finally, through 2,609 related articles reviewing and searching, nine articles were included. The research process was carried out in three centers at Baghdad Medical City including: Baghdad Radiotherapy and Nuclear Medicine Center, Oncology Teaching Hospital, and National Cancer Center at the period from January 2019 to May 2019.

2.2. Study design

We conducted this study under accordance with the preferred reporting items for systematic reviews and meta-analysis (PRISMA) guidelines [19]. We measured the quality of the studies based on the Newcastle–Ottawa Scale that assesses the methodological quality of non-randomised studies for meta-analysis [20]. The scale assessed the selection of studies, and ascertainment of each one. Each positive criterion scores 1 point, with the maximum N-O score is 9.

2.3. Inclusion criteria

1. All English-language articles related to chemoradiation management of rectal cancer.
2. All methods of study, and thesis that associated with the subject of this research.
3. All trials that compare pre- / post-operative chemoradiotherapy.

2.4. Exclusion criteria

1. The non-English-language articles, as were those without full-text access.
2. Scientific documents related to predatory origin.
3. All duplicate articles and records.
4. All literature that the patients presented with colon cancer or anal cancer only.
5. The study was a randomized controlled trial.

2.5. Data sources

The international electronic databases investigated and including English sources from Medline through PubMed, Google Scholar, ResearcGate, Scopus, Embase, ISI Web of Science, Springer databases, ScienceDirect, and the Cochrane Library, were searched and selected. Iraqi Academic Scientific Journals, The Eastern Mediterranean Journals, and African Journals OnLine were also searched for published articles, and other documents were extracted from reports published by organizations.

2.6. Data extraction and collection

The primary data reported included rectal cancer, and patients study characterizes of 101 patients attending Baghdad Medical City Oncology centers. Those, including the gender, age, family history, smoking, comorbidity, IBD, tumor sites, histopathology, stages, grading, distance for anal verge, local recurrence, distant metastasis, type of surgery, chemoradiation details of neoadjuvant and adjuvant therapy. Others for systematic and meta-analysis studies data included time, country, study type, the patients number, treatment types, and year of publication.

2.7. Search strategy

The search for articles was done using a combination of groups of words in the databases mentioned above: rectum (rectal cancer OR rectum tumor OR rectal neoplasm), chemoradiation (chemotherapy OR radiotherapy OR pre-operative OR post-operative OR neoadjuvant OR adjuvant OR chemoradiation OR chemoirradiation OR radio-chemotherapy), surgery (anterior resection of rectum OR total mesorectal excision OR abdominoperineal resection OR anterior resection of rectum), and study (systematic review OR meta-analysis OR cross-sectional OR observational), and (chemoirradiation trials). These groups of words were combined with "AND" together, and used in titles, abstracts, and keywords of used articles.

2.8. Statistical analysis

All data collected were entered statistical analysis into a file of Statistical Package for Social Sciences version 24 (SPSS v24) (SPSS Inc., Chicago, Illinois, USA). Descriptive analysis of clinical and pathological characteristics was performed. A two-sided *P*-value of 0.05 or less was considered statistically significant for Monte Carlo 2-sided Chi-square, and Spearman correlation test. Performed PRISMA flowchart for inclusion and exclusion studies. Assessed the N-O score for including studies with several confounding variables we collected. Forest plots showing comparison between neoadjuvant and adjuvant chemoradiation roles in rectum cancer. A non-random-effects model was used for meta-analysis of all studies by Odds ratios at 95% CI.

Results

3.1. Patients baseline characterizers

Gender distributed as male 49(48.5%), and female 52(51.5%). Regarding the age groups, we recorded 25(24.8%) of patients belonged to 61-70 years, and 20(19.8%), 24(23.8%), 6(5.9%) of them for 41-50 years, 51-60 years, 21-30 years, respectively. Whereas groups 31-40 years, and >70 years presented the same percent of 13(12.9%), with mean±SD = 48.7±14.2 years. Of all 101 patients, there was only 7(6.9%) had a positive family history, while the remaining had a negative family history. Smoker patients in this study were 50(49.5%), yet the non-smoker patients were also presented. The comorbid conditions company rectal cancer found in 46(45.5%), and those free were 55(54.5%). Inflammatory bowel diseases (IBD) were presented in 5(4.9%) patients, whereas the majority were absent as 96(95.1%), as shown in (**Table 1**).

Table 1. Patients baseline characterizers of rectal cancer (n=101).

Characterizes		*n* (%)
Gender	**Male**	49 (48.5)
	Female	52 (51.5)
Age (years) Mean ±SD=**48.7±14.2**	**<20**	0
	21-30	6 (5.9)
	31-40	13 (12.9)
	41-50	20 (19.8)
	51-60	24 (23.8)
	61-70	25 (24.8)
	>70	13 (12.9)
Family history	**Positive**	7 (6.9)
	Negative	94 (93.1)
Smoking	**Smoker**	50 (49.5)
	Non-smoker	51 (50.5)
Comorbidity	**Present**	46 (45.5)
	Absent	55 (54.5)
IBD	**Present**	5 (4.9)
	Absent	96 (95.1)

3.2. Tumor baseline characterizers

The rectosigmoid cancer represented the most common site in this study as 50(49.5%), while rectum, and anorectal were presented as 42(41.6%), and 9(8.9%), respectively. The results showed prominent of adenocarcinoma as most common histopathology as 76(75.2%) of patients. The localized stage of cancer recorded in 50(49.5%) patients, follow regional as 19(18.8%), and metastasis disease in 32(31.7%) of patients. Regarding cancer grading, the moderate differentiation was dominant grade as 65(64.4%), followed by well differentiation 20(19.8%), poorly 14(13.9), and undifferentiated 2(2%). The tumor distant from anal verge results exhibited as <5 cm in 13(12.9%), 5-10 cm in 59(58.4%), and >10 cm in 29(28.7%), as shown in (**Table 2**).

Table 2. Tumor baseline characteristics of rectal cancer (n=101).

Characteristic		*n* (%)
Location	**Rectosigmoid**	50 (49.5)
	Rectum	42 (41.6)
	Anorectal	9 (8.9)
Histopathology	**Adenocarcinoma**	76 (75.2)
	Mucinous carcinoma	13 (12.9)
	Signet-ring cell carcinoma	4 (4)
	Undifferentiated carcinoma	7 (6.9)
	Adenosequomous carcinoma	1(1)
Stages	**Localized**	50 (49.5)
	Regional	19 (18.8)
	Distant Metastasis	32 (31.7)
Grades	**Well differentiation**	20 (19.8)
	Moderate Differentiation	65 (64.4)
	Poorly differentiation	14 (13.9)
	Undifferentiation	2 (2)
Distant from anal verge	**<5 cm**	13 (12.9)
	5-10 cm	59 (58.4)
	>10 cm	29 (28.7)

3.3. Metastasis pattern of rectal cancer

The majority of patients of our study have no metastatic disease as 68(67.3%). Indeed the pulmonary was the most frequent site of distant metastasis that found in 11(10.9%) patients, as well as multiple organs metastasis presented in 10(9.9%) patient. Furthermore, local recurrence found in 7(6.9%) patients, whereas liver and bone secondaries showed the lowest site of metastasis as 2(2%), 3(3%), respectively, as shown in (**Table 3**).

Table 3. Rectal cancer metastasis patterns (n=101).

Characteristic		*n* (%)
Metastatic patterns	**Liver**	2 (2)
	Lung	11 (10.9)
	Local recurrence	7 (6.9)
	Bone	3 (3)
	Multiple metastases	10 (9.9)
	No metastases	68 (67.3)

3.4. Rectal cancer treatment

Most patients undergo different surgical procedures. APR and TME were the prevalent two operations have done in 41(40.6%), 23(22.8%), respectively. Whatever those who have no surgery done for them at all were 25(24.8%). Chemoradiation used in most of the management programs. Adjuvant chemoradiation performed in 40(39.6%), whereas neoadjuvant chemoradiation was given for 25 patients as neoadjuvant chemotherapy+ chemoradiation 12(11.9%), neoadjuvant chemotherapy only 7(6%), and neoadjuvant chemoradiation+ adjuvant chemotherapy 6(5.9%). Radiotherapy or chemotherapy as alone method for treatment, recorded in 4(4%) of patients. Lastly, palliation modalities were used in 32(31.7%) of patients, as shown in (**Table 4**).

Table 4. Rectal cancer management (n=101).

Variables		*n* (%)
Surgery	**APR**	41 (40.6)
	LAR+ loop ieliostomy	4 (4)
	LAR without ieliostomy	3 (3)
	TME	23 (22.8)
	Local excision	5 (5)
	***No* surgery**	25 (24.8)
Chemoradiation	**Neoadjuvant chemotherapy + Chemoradiation**	12 (11.9)
	Neoadjuvant RT+ Adjuvant chemotherapy	4 (4)
	Neoadjuvant chemoradiation	7 (6.9)
	Neoadjuvant chemoradiation + Adjuvant chemotherapy	6 (5.9)
	Adjuvant chemoradiation	40 (39.6)
	Palliative chemoradiation	32 (31.7)

3.5. Correlation results of the study

All crossing relation between cancer staging and surgical operation types demonstrated significant correlation (x^2=8.89, *r*=0.001, *P*=0.018), mostly among localized disease undergo local excision 24(23.8%), metastatic cancer with APR 20(19.8%), and those have localized stages operated by TME 14(13.9%). We obtained a substantial significant differences (x^2=54.1, *r*=0.726, *P*<0.0001), between chemoradiation regimens and staging, which more noticed among localized stages received adjuvant chemoradiation 30(29.7%), and patients have metastasis given palliative chemoradiation 32(31.7%), as shown in (**Table 5**).

Tumor grading had a significant association for management modalities in our study, which illustrated in (**Table 6**). As a result cancer stages have significant difference among surgery methods (x^2=1.61, *r*=0.07, *P*=0.041), seen mostly in moderately differentiated grade as 20(19.8%) of patients undergo local excision,

21(20.8%) patients treated by APR, and 14(13.9%) operated by TME. Regarding chemoradiation and grading showed a statistical significant (x^2=8.55, *r*=0.298, *P*=0.016), mostly on moderate grading treated by adjuvant and palliative chemotherapy, as 26(25.7%), 25(24.8%), respectively.

In addition the histopathology of rectal cancer have significant correlation for both surgical operations (x^2=1.006, *r*=0.078, *P*=0.013), and chemoradiation (x^2=4.055, *r*=0.095, *P*=0.025). Adenocarcinoma mostly mirrored this relation in patients undergo local excision 26(25.7%), AR 23(22.7%), and TME 17(16.8%), and as well as for those received adjuvant or palliative chemoradiation, as 29(28.7%), 23(22.8%), respectively, as showed in (**Table 7**).

The distance from anal verge, and the 5-10 cm mostly, showed a significant differences for surgical operations (x^2=1.044, *r*=0.055, *P*=0.012), especially for those who undergo local excision 28(27.7%), and the chemoradiation protocols (x^2=1.255, *r*=0.14, *P*=0.014), which mostly among patients received adjuvant chemoradiation 26(25.7%), as shown in (**Table 8**).

Lastly, the rectal cancer sites, mostly rectosigmoid, and rectum displayed a significant association for surgical operations (x^2=1.7, *r*=0.012, *P*=0.045), for those have rectosigmoid treated with local excision 14(13.9%), TME 12(11.8%), and APR 18(17.9%), and for rectum undergo local excision 16(15.8%). The crossing with chemoradiation more seen in recto-sigmoid cancer among adjuvant chemoradiation 19(18.8%), and palliative chemoradiation 18(17.8%), as well as in rectum cancer received adjuvant treatment 17(16.8%), which exhibited a significant differences (x^2=2.7, *r*=0.052, *P*=0.05), as shown in (**Table 9**).

Table 5. Tumor staging crossing treatment options of rectal cancer.

Variables		Stages			Monte Carlo x^2 test	Spearman correlation (*r*)	*P* value
		Localized	**Regional**	**Distant metastases**			
		***n*(%)**					
Surgery	**APR**	10 (9.8)	5 (5)	20 (19.8)	8.98	0.001	0.018
	LAR+ loop ieliostomy	1 (1)	0	3 (3)			
	LAR without ieliostomy	1 (1)	1 (1)	1 (1)			
	TME	14 (13.9)	8 (7.9)	1 (1)			
	Local excision	24 (23.8)	5 (5)	2 (2)			
CRT	**Neoadjuvant chemotherapy + CRT**	8 (7.9)	4 (4)	0	54.1	0.726	<0.0001
	Neoadjuvant RT+ Adjuvant chemotherapy	2 (2)	2 (2)	0			
	Neoadjuvant CRT	6 (5.9)	1 (1)	0			
	Neoadjuvant CRT + Adjuvant chemotherapy	4 (4)	2 (2)	0			
	Adjuvant CRT	30 (29.7)	10 (9.9)	0			
	Palliative CRT	0	0	32 (31.7)			

Table 6. Tumor grading correlation to management modalities of rectal cancer.

Variables		Grades				Monte Carlo x^2 test	Spearman correlation (r)	***P* value**
		Well differentiation	**Moderate differentiation**	**Poorly differentiation**	**Undifferentiation**			
		***n*(%)**						
Surgery	**APR**	5 (5)	21 (20.8)	8 (7.9)	2 (2)	1.61	0.07	0.041
	LAR+ loop ieliostomy	0	4 (4)	0	0			
	LAR without ieliostomy	0	3 (3)	0	0			
	TME	7 (6.9)	14 (13.9)	2 (2)	0			
	Local excision	7 (6.9)	20 (19.8)	3 (3)	1 (1)			
CRT	**Neoadjuvant chemotherapy + CRT**	8 (7.9)	3 (3)	1 (1)	0	8.55	0.298	0.016
	Neoadjuvant RT+ Adjuvant chemotherapy	1 (1)	3 (3)	0	0			
	Neoadjuvant CRT	1 (1)	4 (4)	2 (2)	0			
	Neoadjuvant CRT + Adjuvant chemotherapy	1 (1)	4 (4)	1 (1)	0			
	Adjuvant CRT	8 (7.9)	26 (25.7)	4 (4)	2 (2)			
	Palliative CRT	1 (1)	25 (24.8)	6 (5.9)	0			

Table 7. Tumor histopathology crossing management options of rectal cancer.

Variables		Histopathology					Monte Carlo x^2 test	Spearman correlation (r)	P value
		Adenocarcinoma	Mucinous carcinoma	Signet-ring cell carcinoma	Undifferentiated carcinoma	Adenosequomous carcinoma			
		$n(\%)$							
Surgery	**APR**	23 (22.7)	5 (5)	2 (2)	4 (4)	0	1.006	0.078	0.013
	LAR+ loop ieliostomy	3 (3)	1 (1)	0	0	0			
	LAR without ieliostomy	3 (3)	0	0	0	0			
	TME	17 (16.8)	3 (3)	2 (2)	1 (1)	0			
	Local excision	26 (25.7)	3 (3)	0	1 (1)	1 (1)			
CRT	**Neoadjuvant chemotherapy + CRT**	10 (9.9)	1 (1)	1 (1)	0	0	4.055	0.095	0.025
	Neoadjuvant RT+ Adjuvant chemotherapy	4 (4)	0	0	0	0			
	Neoadjuvant CRT	6 (5.9)	0	0	1 (1)	0			
	Neoadjuvant CRT + Adjuvant chemotherapy	4 (4)	1 (1)	0	1 (1)	0			
	Adjuvant CRT	29 (28.7)	6 (5.9)	1 (1)	3 (3)	1 (1)			
	Palliative CRT	23 (22.8)	5 (5)	2 (2)	2 (2)	0			

Table 8. Distance from anal verge crossing management options of rectal cancer.

Variables		Distance from anal verge			Monte Carlo x^2 test	Spearman correlation (*r*)	***P* value**
		< 5 cm	**5-10 cm**	**> 10 cm**			
			***n*(%)**				
Surgery	**APR**	12 (11.9)	13 (12.9)	10 (9.9)	1.044	0.055	0.012
	LAR+ loop ieliostomy	0	2 (2)	2 (2)			
	LAR without ieliostomy	0	1 (1)	2 (2)			
	TME	0	13 (12.9)	10 (9.9)			
	Local excision	0	28 (27.7)	3 (3)			
CRT	**Neoadjuvant chemotherapy + CRT**	1 (1)	7 (6.9)	4 (4)	1.255	0.14	0.014
	Neoadjuvant RT+ Adjuvant chemotherapy	1 (1)	2 (2)	1 (1)			
	Neoadjuvant CRT	1 (1)	5 (5)	1 (1)			
	Neoadjuvant CRT + Adjuvant chemotherapy	1 (1)	5 (5)	0			
	Adjuvant CRT	5 (5)	26 (25.7)	9 (8.9)			
	Palliative CRT	4 (4)	14 (13.9)	14 (13.9)			

Table 9. Tumor sites crossing management options of rectal cancer.

Variables		Sites			Monte Carlo x^2 test	Spearman correlation (*r*)	*P* value
		Recto-sigmoid	**Rectum**	**Anorectal**			
		***n*(%)**					
Surgery	**APR**	18 (17.9)	13 (12.9)	4 (4)	1.7	0.012	0.045
	LAR+ loop ieliostomy	3 (3)	1 (1)	0			
	LAR without ieliostomy	2 (2)	1 (1)	0			
	TME	12 (11.9)	8 (7.9)	3 (3)			
	Local excision	14 (13.9)	16 (15.8)	1 (1)			
CRT	**Neoadjuvant chemotherapy + CRT**	6 (5.9)	6 (5.9)	0	2.7	0.052	0.05
	Neoadjuvant RT+ Adjuvant chemotherapy	2 (2)	2 (2)	0			
	Neoadjuvant CRT	3 (3)	4 (4)	0			
	Neoadjuvant CRT + Adjuvant chemotherapy	2 (2)	2 (2)	2 (2)			
	Adjuvant CRT	19 (18.8)	17 (16.8)	4 (4)			
	Palliative CRT	18 (17.8)	11 (10.9)	3 (3)			

3.6. Meta-analysis findings

A total of 2,609 articles with 1,377 citations from 12 databases met our search strategies about rectal cancer were searched from 2015 to 2019. Duplication screening done resulted in 789 articles were excluded after reviewing of titles/abstracts. Then 132 articles retrieved after the second review. In the full articles text screen a total of 356 article were excluded. Also, during the process of data extraction, 91 articles were excluded. Finally, Nine studies were included in a meta-analysis of our study after reviewing of the full-text articles that adequately match the inclusion and exclusion criteria (**All references listed in the appendix**), as shown in (**Figure 1**).

The highest Newcastle-Ottawa score (8) demonstrated in three studies, which were Ellis 2019; Spiegel 2018; Mancini 2017, whereas median score (7) calculated in five studies, they were Chapman 2019; Quezada-Diaz 2019; Franke 2017; Dossa 2017; Rodel 2016. Lastly, the low score (6) obtained in Kimberly 2017 only, as showed in (**Table 10**).

All nine articles described chemoradiation as the main subject in the management of rectal cancer. Three articles conducted in 2019 by Ellis CT; Chapman W; Quezada-Diaz F, one in 2018 by Spiegel D, four in 2017 by Mancini R; Franke AJ; Dossa F; Kimberly P, and one in 2016 by Rodel C, as shown in (**Table 11**).

Different study models used, different sample size, and period. Comparison, cohort, systematic review, analysis, meta-analysis, and randomized studies were thoroughly reviewed in details. Many outcomes obtained range from the complete response, improvement in OS, DFS, and LR. Most of the patients in nine studies undergo TME as the main surgical operation (**Table 11**). Forest plots showing chemoradiation roles in rectum cancer, with overall shifted to neoadjuvant side at heterogeneity was I^2 = 73.1; P= 0.001. A non-random-effects model was used for meta-analysis by Odds ratios of each studies at 95%CI (**Figure 2**).

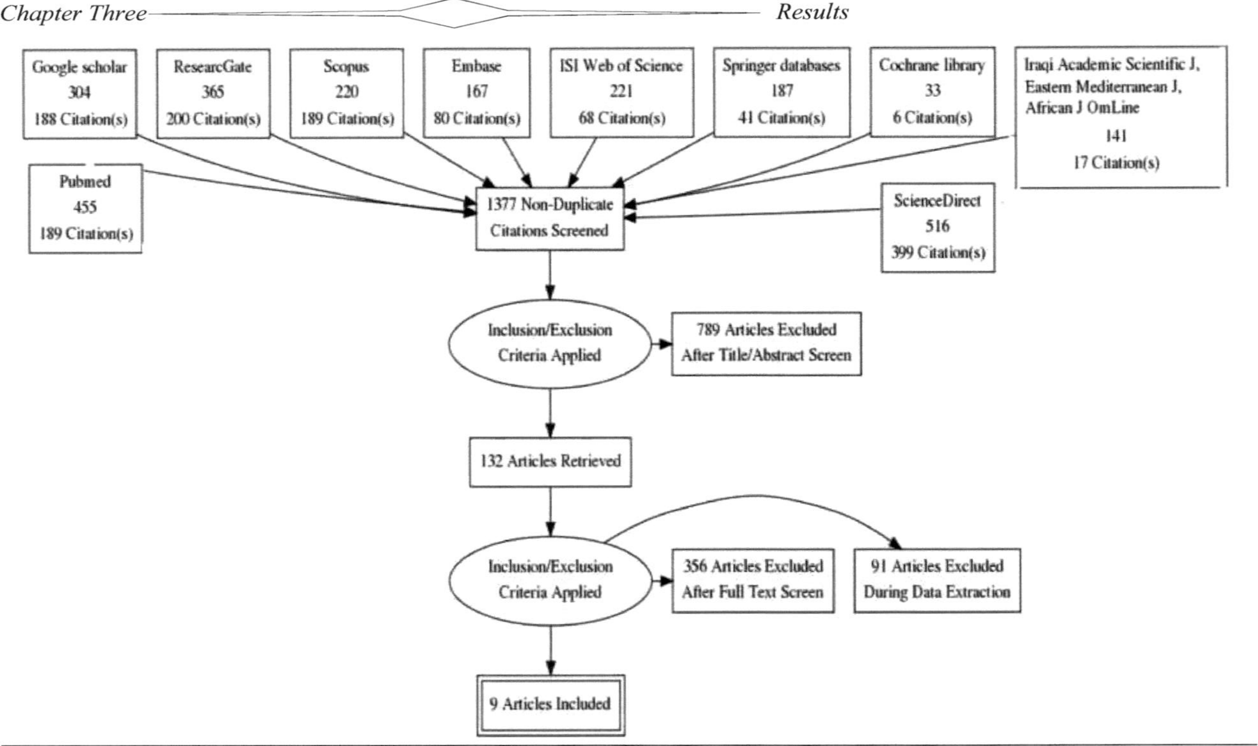

Figure 1. PRISMA flowchart to include and exclude articles of chemoradiation roles in the management of rectal cancer in this study

Table 10. Newcastle–Ottawa scale of the eligible nine studies.

	Newcastle–Ottawa scale								
Study ID	Is the definition adequate?	Is it representative?	Selection adequate	Definition of meta-analysis	Study for the most important	Study for Important Additional	Ascertainment adequate	Same method of ascertainment	Non-rcsponse rate adequate	Total score /9
Ellis 2019	yes	yes	yes	yes	yes	yes	unclear	yes	yes	8
Chapman 2019	yes	yes	unclear	yes	yes	yes	yes	unclear	yes	7
Quezada-Diaz 2019	yes	yes	unclear	yes	yes	yes	yes	yes	no	7
Spiegel 2018	yes	yes	yes	yes	yes	no	yes	yes	yes	8
Mancini 2017	yes	yes	yes	no	yes	yes	yes	yes	yes	8
Franke 2017	yes	yes	yes	no	yes	yes	yes	yes	unclear	7
Dossa 2017	yes	yes	yes	yes	yes	yes	unclear	yes	unclear	7
Kimberly 2017	yes	yes	yes	no	no	yes	yes	yes	unclear	6
Rodel 2016	yes	yes	yes	yes	yes	yes	unclear	yes	unclear	7

Table 11. Meta-analysis of the eligible nine studies.

Study	Type	*n* of patients	Chemoradiation	Follow up period	Outcome	Conclusions	N–O Score
Ellis et al, 2019	Comparison SEER-Medicare	482	Adjuvant / neoadjuvant plus surgery	24 month	2.5% / 3.4% complete response	Treated with CRT-only were less likely to receive surveillance than those treated with conventional treatment	8
Chapman et al, 2019	Retrospective cohort study	388	Neoadjuvant, and TME	9 years	pCR rate of 25% and overall recurrence rate of 14.9%	Short course radiation with neoadjuvant multi-agent chemotherapy is at least as effective as long-course CRT	7
Quezada-Diaz et al, 2019	Retrospective review	176	Adjuvant, neoadjuvant, and surgery	6 years	-	The trimodality treatment does not seem to impair bowel function	7
Spiegel et al, 2018	Veterans Health Administration analysis	649	Adjuvant, neoadjuvant, and TMR	66 months	Improve both OS and DFS	There was no improvement in OS or DFS with the addition of a multi-agent over single-agent chemotherapy	8
Mancini et al, 2017	Multiple correspondence analysis	174	Neoadjuvant plus surgery	10 years	13.2% complete response	Neoadjuvant CRT and radical surgery enrich the prognostic profile of patients	8
Franke et al, 2017	Systematic review	-	Neoadjuvant plus surgery	5 years	Reduced local recurrence rates	Outline the pragmatic opportunities for future investigation into questions of efficacy, safety, and ultimate improvements	7
Dossa et	Systematic	867	Neoadjuvant	12-68	-	Most patients treated by	7

al, 2017	review and meta-analysis		plus watch-and-wait	months		watch-and-wait avoid radical surgery and of those who have regrowth almost all have salvage therapy	
Kimberly et al, 2017	Phase II randomized trial	93	Adjuvant and neoadjuvant plus surgery	4 years	All patients had resolution of bleeding and improvement of obstructive symptoms, with no complications requiring surgical intervention.	TRIAL seems to be a well-tolerated alternative to the current standard treatment sequence.	6
Rodel et al, 2016	Meta-analysis	-	Preoperative / postoperative plus TME	-	Encouraging pCR rates but increased surgical complications	The benefit role of induction and consolidation chemotherapy before or after CRT. The minimal or omitted surgery following complete response to CRT The omission of radiotherapy for selected patients with response to neoadjuvant chemotherapy.	7

CRT, chemoradiation; pCR, pathological complete response; OS, overall survival; DFS, disease free survival; TMR, total mesorectal excision; N-O, Newcastle–Ottawa

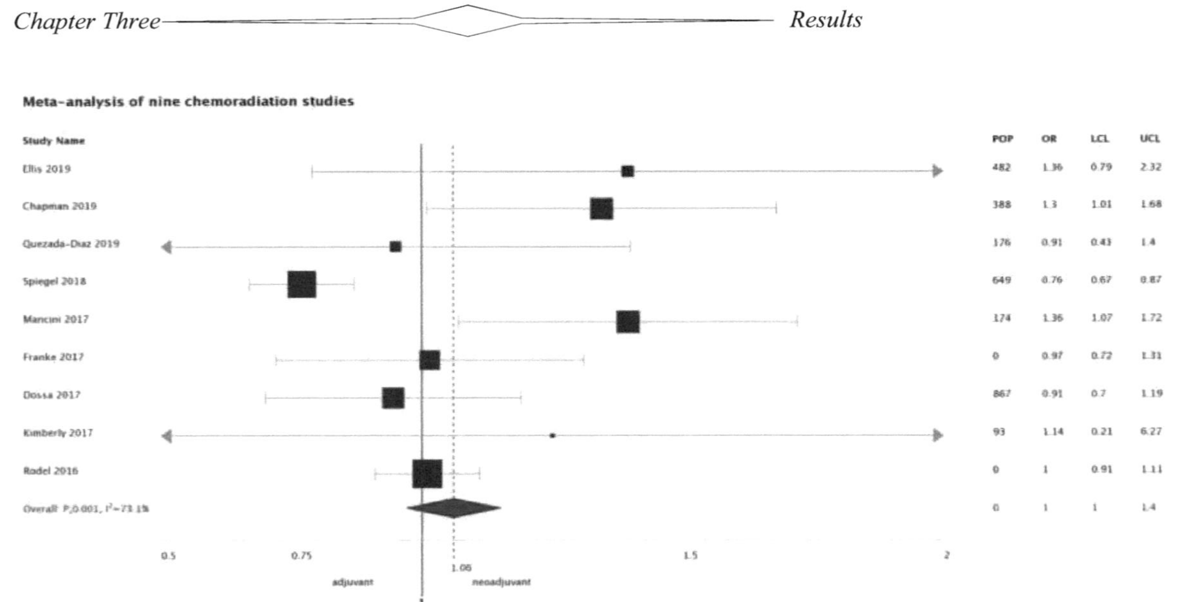

Figure 2. Forest plot showing chemoradiation roles in rectum cancer. A non-random-effects model was used for meta-analysis. Odds ratios are shown with 95%CI.

Discussion

Our findings regarding gender estimated 49(48.5%) were men, and 52(51.5%) were women. Similarly, results were reported by Radhi et al., 2018 in Al-Diwaniyah [21], Alsafi et al., 2018 in Karbala [22], whereas different from studies conducted in Misan by Alhilfi et al., 2019 [23], and Khalil et al., 2018 in Duhok [24]. A report registered in the Iraqi cancer registry for the period 2002-2011 and in the National Cancer Hospitals between 2012 and 2014, found that male to female ratio varied from 1.17:1 to 1.28:1 [25].

Belong to the age groups, the peak incidences were found in 25(24.8%) of patients to 61-70 years, and 24(23.8%) of patients to 51-60 years. These findings, like many data reported by studies in our country and worldwide status [1, 5, 8-10, 20-28]. Age is an essential factor for the occurrence and management of rectal cancer [6, 26].

Of all 101 patients, there was only 7(6.9%) had a positive family history, while the remaining had negative family history as 94(93.1%). Tobacco smoking as a risk factor presented in 50(49.5%) of patients. The comorbid conditions company rectal cancer found in 46(45.5%). Furthermore, the IBD was presented in 5(4.9%) patients only. Many factors shown to increase the risk of developing colorectal cancer including: increasing age; male sex; family history; inflammatory bowel disease; increasing height; increasing body mass index; consumption of processed meat, refined grains, starches, and sugars; excessive alcohol intake and smoking; and low folate consumption [1, 4-6, 8-10]. Of these, only increasing age, male sex, and excessive alcohol use have been associated with rectal cancer [26].

The tumor characteristics in this study revealed that rectosigmoid cancer represented the most current site as 50(49.5%) of patients, while rectum, and anorectal were presented as 42(41.6%), and 9(8.9%), respectively. This information resembling many studies outside Iraq [27, 28], whereas disagreeing with Radhi et al., 2018 [21], Alsafi et al., 2018 [22], Alhilfi et al., 2019 [23], and Khalil et al., 2018 [24] studies. Those may be estimated the non-real figures because of many patients prefer to do a colonoscopy in the different provinces and even outside the country, besides that many cases of rectal cancer diagnosed by imaging studies such as CT scan or the US and undergo surgery without doing colonoscopy or sigmoidoscopy.

On the other hand, we received many cases for colonoscopy referred to the center from other provinces so that figures may not reflect the distribution of the disease site or locations. The highest recto-sigmoid cancer incidence rates are found in Europe (eg, Hungary, Slovenia, Slovakia, the Netherlands, and Norway), Australia/New Zealand, Northern America, and Eastern Asia (Japan and the Republic of Korea, Singapore [in females]), with Hungary and Norway, rates also are elevated in Uruguay among both men and women. Rectal cancer incidence rates have a similar regional distribution, although the highest rates are seen in the Republic of Korea among males and Macedonia among females. Rates of both colon and rectal cancer incidence tend to be low in most regions of Africa and Southern Asia [4, 10].

The results showed prominent of adenocarcinoma as most common histopathology as 76(75.2%) of patients. The localized stage without metastasis of cancer recorded in 50(49.5%) patients, while metastasis disease observed in 32(31.7%) of patients. Regarding cancer grading, the moderate differentiation was dominant grade as 65(64.4%), followed by well differentiation 20(19.8%), poorly 14(13.9), and undifferentiated 2(2%). Tumors of the rectum arise in the mucosa, and virtually all (>90%) are adenocarcinomas [26]. Other histologic types include squamous cell carcinoma, melanoma, small-cell carcinoma, carcinoid, sarcoma, and lymphoma in different proportions. Most grading systems classify adenocarcinoma as well, moderately or poorly differentiated [6, 8, 10, 26]. All studies conducted in various provinces in our countries demonstrated the same results [2, 20-25].

Mostly, the 5-10 cm distant of tumor from the anal verge was the common finding exhibited as 59(58.4%) of patients. Khan et al., concluded that the distance of rectal cancer from the anal verge influenced the use of neoadjuvant treatment and ultimate R0 resection rate [29]. The tumor location and the distal tumor margin are essential factors upon which the surgical plan for patients with rectal cancer is based. Accurate measurement of the distal tumor margin is necessary in planning the surgical procedure, even sphincter-saving resection [29].

The pulmonary site was most frequent site of distant metastasis that found in 11(10.9%) patients, as well as multiple organs metastasis presented in 10(9.9%) patient. Furthermore, local recurrence found in 7(6.9%) patients, whereas liver and bone secondaries showed the lowest site of metastasis as 2(2%), 3(3%), respectively. Large-bowel tumors invading from mucosa through the wall and beyond that, with the involvement of lymphatic vessels and lymph nodes, as well as the hematogenous spread can occur, primarily to the lung and liver [26]. Pulmonary metastasis occurred more frequently in patients with lower rectal cancer than in those with upper rectal cancer [10, 26]. Metastases to the regional lymph nodes are found in 40% to 70% of cases at the time of resection. Venous or lymphatic invasion is found in up to 60% of cases. Rectal cancers are three times more likely to recur locally than are proximal colonic tumors, because the anatomic confine of the rectum precludes wide resection margins, and the rectum lacks an outer serosal layer through most of its course. Due to the venous and lymphatic drainage of the rectum go to the inferior vena cava, it has a higher incidence of lung metastasis compared with colon cancers that more frequently recurs first in the liver [1, 6, 8, 10, 26].

Information regarding types of surgery were inadequate in Iraq due to inadequate surgical reports written by surgeons. Many surgical procedures perform for rectal cancer as Hartmann procedure, total procto-coloctomy, anterior resection, APR, and ileal pouch - anastomosis. Most patients of our study undergo APR and TME operations, were the most prevalent two procedures have done in 41(40.6%), 23(22.8%), respectively. Chemoradiation used in most of management modalities. Adjuvant chemoradiation performed in 40(39.6%), whereas neoadjuvant chemoradiation was given for 25 patients as neoadjuvant chemotherapy+ chemoradiation 12(11.9%), neoadjuvant chemotherapy only 7(6%), and neoadjuvant chemoradiation+ adjuvant chemotherapy 6(5.9%). Radiotherapy or chemotherapy as alone method for treatment, recorded in 4(4%) of patients. Lastly, palliation modalities were used in 32(31.7%) of patients.

All relation between cancer staging, surgical operations, and chemoradiation demonstrated significant differences (x^2=8.89, r=0.001, P=0.018), (x^2=54.1, r=0.726, P<0.0001), respectively. The grading had significant association for management modalities in our study, (x^2=1.61, r=0.07, P=0.041), and (x^2=8.55, r=0.298, P=0.016), respectively. In addition the histopathology of rectal cancer have significant correlation for both surgical operations (x^2=1.006, r=0.078, P=0.013), and chemoradiation (x^2=4.055, r=0.095, P=0.025). The distance form anal verge, and the 5-10 cm mostly, showed a significant differences for surgical operations (x^2=1.044, r=0.055, P=0.012), and the chemoradiation protocols (x^2=1.255, r=0.14, P=0.014). The rectal cancer sites, mostly rectosigmoid, and rectum displayed a significant association for surgical operations (x^2=1.7, r=0.012, P=0.045), and with chemoradiation (x^2=2.7, r=0.052, P=0.05).

Most trails and studies conducting to demonstrate good outcomes of chemoradiation in rectal cancer have a significant improvement in survival and patient quality life. The GITSG 7175 reported that chemoradiation arm improved 5-year DFS and OS over control [8-10].

The National Cancer Institute (NCI) and Mayo/NCCTG 79-47-51 concluded that chemoradiation was the standard postoperative adjuvant treatment for all patients with pT3 or N1-2 disease, and demonstrated improvements in both DFS and OS [11].

The NSABP R-01, R-02 reported rectal cancer with B-C (II-III) treated with surgery alone vs. post-op RT vs. post-op chemo. RT improved LF (25 vs16%), while chemo improved DFS (30 vs 42%) and OS (43 vs 53%) vs. observation [6, 8-10].

EORTC trial 22921 is found a significant decrease in the local failure rate in those patients who receive chemoradiation compared with irradiation (8% to 10% versus 17%; $p < 0.001$) but no difference in the 5-year OS (65%) [12].

The NSABP R0-354 and the German CAO/ ARO/AIO 94 trials are based on pilot data suggesting that chemotherapy increased the response rate of preoperative radiation, and because of less small bowel in the radiation field, the acute toxicity of preoperative chemoradiation was less then postoperative chemoradiation [14].

The STAR-01, ACCORD, and NSABP R-04 trials, shown a significant improvement in pCR (17% versus 13%, $p = 0.045$) with no corresponding increase in acute grade 3+ toxicity (23% versus 22%) [15, 16].

The UK MRC CR07 trial (short course) randomized patients with clinical stages I to III rectal cancer to preoperative irradiation or selective postoperative chemoradiation, the patients who received preoperative had significantly lower 3-year local recurrence rates (4.4% versus 10.6%; $p < 0.0001$) [15]. The short-course radiation (25 Gy in 5 fractions) is established in the Dutch Colorectal Cancer Group CKVO, and Swedish Rectal Cancer trials and chemoradiation is established by the German Rectal Cancer Trial CAO/ARO/ AIO-94 (45-50.4 Gy in 25 to 28 fractions plus concurrent chemotherapy) [15-17]. Polish Colorectal Study Group trial randomized patients with cT3 rectal cancers to preoperative short-course radiation compared to chemoradiation [10]. This showed a higher pCR rate (16% versus 1%) and a lower incidence of positive radial margins (4% versus 13%, $p = 0.017$) [17]. Pooled-analysis on NCCTG trials, Int 0144, NSABP RO1, and RO2, revealed that post-op chemo appeared to improve OS, similar to post-op chemoradiation, but the DFS, OS, and LF tended to be better with chemoradiation [18].

The present meta-analysis demonstrates a significant reduction in local recurrence rate with the addition of chemotherapy over all nine studies. Importantly, the cumulative incidence rates of local recurrence in the RT group of the studies were (17%) and in both groups of the study (15%) seem high compared to the 5.5% local recurrence rate at 5 years achieved by the Dutch rectal cancer trial using preoperative RT followed by surgery [11, 14]. Differences in stage distribution and variation in surgical technique might be the cause. Indeed, during the Dutch rectal cancer trial, a formal surgical training and quality control program was implemented to guarantee optimal surgery TME [10, 11].

Although in the studies of 2017 by Mancini et al; Franke et al; Dossa et al; Kimberly et al, a marginally significant five year survival benefit were associated with CRT, the combined analysis resulted in demonstrating a significant difference in either OS or DFS.

This formulated as a novel point of our study to explain that survival benefit found in many pre or postoperative adjuvant therapy trials in rectal cancer. But, we have argued that the follow-up time of our study is too short to observe a survival benefit, or that the incidence of local recurrence is too low to influence survival. However, chemotherapy-related toxicity was generally acceptable, as evidenced by the high compliance rates in all studies mentioned.

The results of this meta-analysis confirm the enhanced antitumor efficacy of combined RT with chemotherapy. Also showed that compared to preoperative RT alone, preoperative CRT improves local control in resectable rectal cancer.

Those represent the novel findings of our study, which are primarily described as the first study done in Iraq, other novelty that the description of a significant association between most of the tumor characters and management multimodalities. Besides that, our findings were more significant supportive of the highest benefits from chemoradiation in the management of rectal cancer.

The role of neoadjuvant CRT before radical surgery is to delay the development of pelvic recurrence of rectal cancer, in the other word to decrease failure rate, also it will cause down- staging or down- sizing of tumor lead to feasible get close circumferential resection margin, enhance effectiveness in well oxygenation of tissue for repair, and save anal sphincter preservation.

When add chemotherapy to radiotherapy, this drug act as radiosensitizer to increase radiotherapy effect on primary tumor, so this may cause complete sterilized of this tumor after complete resection, but here still micro - metastatic cells may not die, so the role of adjuvant chemotherapy required.

The time between CRT and surgery very important issue for get more complete response from cancer management. The preoperative CRT may increase the rate of pathological complete response but can't improve disease free survival (DFS) or overall survival (OS) significantly. Whereas, there are improvement in local control but at the expense of treatment related toxicities and not effect sphincter preservation with long term survival.

There are some limitations we noticed about this study as short time to conduct such study beside difficulty in emerging follow up for the patients included due to short time.

Here all patients are electively included as we deal with those who received CRT in our centers, but due to that a lot of patients may be the majority that discovered to have rectosigmoid tumor as emergency intestinal obstructions were hidden or missing.

1. Conclusions

1. The incidence of rectal cancer is mostly belongs to 5th, and 6th decade of life.
2. The family history, tobacco smoking, comorbid conditions, and the IBD behave unmarked effect as risk factors.
3. Rectosigmoid cancer represents the most common site, follow by rectum, with prominent of adenocarcinoma as most common histopathology, and of moderate differentiation grade.
4. Mostly, the 5-10 cm distant of tumor from anal verge was the common finding exhibited, and this importantly in influenced the use of neoadjuvant treatment and planning the surgical procedure.
5. The pulmonary was most typical site of distant metastasis followed by multiple organs metastasis.
6. All relation between cancer characters, surgical operations, and chemoradiation demonstrated significant differences.
7. We meta-analyzed a significant reduction in local recurrence rate with the addition of chemotherapy to radiotherapy.
8. The formulated a novel point that survival benefit found in many pre or postoperative chemoradiation trials in rectal cancer.

2. Recommendations

1. All results support need more studies conduction using the same design for different cancer types in the future, beside this, giving more accurate information than simple observational studies.
2. Future designing such study in many subjects of clinical oncology because it may be equal to a randomized trial in its efficacy and building up.
3. The requirement for more time to conduct similar studies, since the time of follow up is the major limitation.

References

1. **Minsky BD, Rodel CM, Valentini V (2016).** In: Gunderson and Tepper (editors). Clinical Radiation Oncology: Rectal cancer, overview. 4th edt. Netherlands, Elsevier, Inc.p:992-1017.
2. **Iraqi Cancer Registry (2011).** Ministry Of Health, Iraqi Cancer Board, Baghdad, Iraq. https://moh.gov.iq/upload/upfile/ar/273.pdf.
3. **Iraqi Cancer Registry (2015).** Annual Report. Iraqi Cancer Registry Board, Ministry Of Health and Environment. Baghdad, Iraq.
4. **Bray F, Ferlay J, Soerjomataram I, et al., (2018).** Global Cancer Statistics 2018: GLOBOCAN Estimates of Incidence and Mortality Worldwide for 36 Cancers in 185 Countries. CA CANCER J CLIN;68:394–424.
5. **NCCN (2019).** Clinical Practice Guidelines in Oncology. Rectal Cancer Version.2. www.nccn.org.
6. **Alberts SR, Grothy A (2012).** In: Casciato DA and Territo MC (editors). Manual of Clinical Oncology: Colorectal cancer. 7th edt. Lippincott Williams & Wilkins, a Wolters Kluwer business. USA. 2012. p:239-258.
7. **Mathis KL, Nelson H, Pemberton JH, et al., (2009).** Un-resectable colorectal cancer can be cured with multimodality therapy. Ann Surg 248:592–598.
8. **Nash MB, Chung HT, Kavita K (2010).** In: Hansen RK and Roach III M (editors). Handbook of Evidence-Based Radiation Oncology: Colorectal cancer. 2nd ed. Springer Science+Business Media, LLC. CA. USA. p:381-390.
9. **Minsky BD (2004).** In: Leibel SA, Phillips TL, editors. Textbook of radiation oncology: Cancer of the Rectum. 2nd ed. Philadelphia: Saunders; p:897-912.
10. **Mohiuddin M, Willett CG (2015).** In: Halperin EC, Perez CA, Brady LW, et al., (editors). Principles and practice of radiation oncology: Colon and Rectum. 6th ed. Philadelphia: Lippincott Williams & Wilkins; p:1366-1382.

11. **Collette L, Bosset JF, den Dulk M, et al., (2007).** Patients with curative resection of cT3-4 rectal cancer after preoperative radiotherapy or radiochemotherapy: Does anybody benefit from adjuvant fluorouracil-based chemotherapy? A trial of the European Organisation for Research and Treatment of Cancer Radiation Oncology Group. J Clin Oncol 25:4379–4386.

12. **Bosset JF, Calais G, Mineur L, et al., (2014).** Fluorouracil-based adjuvant chemotherapy after preoperative chemoradiotherapy in rectal cancer: Long-term results of the EORTC 22921 randomised study. Lancet Oncol 15:184–190.

13. **Gerard JP, Conroy T, Bonnetain F (2006).** Preoperative radiotherapy with or without concurrent fluorouracil and leucovorin in T3-4 rectal cancers: Results of FFCD 9203. J Clin Oncol 28:4620–4625.

14. **Sauer R, Liersch T, Merkel S, et al., (2012).** Preoperative versus postoperative chemoradiotherapy for locally advanced rectal cancer: Results of the German CAO/ARO/AIO-94 randomized phase III trial after a median follow-up of 11 years. J Clin Oncol 30:1926–1933.

15. **Quirke P, Steele R, Monson J, et al., (2009).** Effect of the plane of surgery achieved on local recurrence in patients with operable rectal cancer: A prospective study using data from the MRC CR07 and NCIC-CTG Co16 randomised clinical trial. Lancet 373:821–828.

16. **Bosset JF, Collette L, Bardet E, et al., (2006).** Chemotherapy with preoperative radiotherapy in rectal cancer. New Engl J Med 355:1114–1123.

17. **Smalley SR, Benedetti JK, Williamson SK, et al., (2006).** Phase III trial of fluorouracil-based chemotherapy regimens plus radiotherapy in postoperative adjuvant rectal cancer: GI INT 0144. J Clin Oncol 24:3542–3547.

18. **Gunderson LL, Sargent D, Tepper JE, et al., (2004).** Impact of T and N stage and treatment on survival and relapse in adjuvant rectal cancer: A pooled analysis. J Clin Oncol 22:1785–1796.

19.**Moher D, Liberati A, Tetzlaff J, et al., (2009).** Preferred reporting items for systematic reviews and meta-analyses: the PRISMA statement. PLoS Med. 6(7):e1000097.

20.**Wells GA, Shea B, O'Connell D, et al., (2019).** The Newcastle-Ottawa Scale (NOS) for assessing the quality of non-randomised studies in meta-analyses. Ottawa Hospital Research Institute. http://www.ohri.ca/programs/ clinical_epidemiology / oxford.asp

21.**Radhi AA, Muslim OT, Abdlmaged MA (2018).** Epidemiological distribution of colorectal cancer in AL-Diwaniyah province, Iraq: an observational study. J Pharm Sci & Res.10(7):1758-1760.

22.**AlSafi RAR, Metib NJ, Hameedi AD et al., (2018).** The Clinical and Pathological Characteristics of Colorectal Cancer in Young Age Group in Karbala Province/ Iraq. Karbala J Med. 11(2):4025-4031.

23.**Alhilfi HSQ, Almohammadawi KOM, Alsaad RKA et al., (2019).** Colorectal cancer epidemiology and clinical study in Misan. Journal of Coloproctology (RIO J). 39(2):159-162.

24.**Khalil KH, Al-Hassawi BA, Abdo JM (2018).** Histopathological evaluation of colorectal carcinoma. Duhok Medical Journal. 12(2):45-68.

25.**Al-Dahhan SA, Al-Lami FH (2018).** Epidemiology of Colorectal Cancer in Iraq, 2002-2014. Gulf J Oncolog. 1(26):23-26.

26.**Palta M, Willett CG, Czito BG (2013).** In: Halperin EC, Perez CA, Brady LW, et al., (editors). Principles and practice of radiation oncology: Cancer of the Colon and Rectum. 6th ed. Philadelphia: Lippincott Williams & Wilkins; p:1215-1230.

27.**Siegel R, Ma J, Zou Z, et al., (2014).** Cancer statistics, 2014. CA Cancer J Clin 64:9–29.

28.**SEER (2014).** Surveillance, Epidemiology, and End Results. Stat Fact Sheets: Rectal Cancer. Archived from the original on 3 July 2014. Retrieved 18 June 2014. https://seer.cancer.gov.

29. **Khan MAS, Ang CW, Hakeem AR (2017).** The Impact of Tumour Distance From the Anal Verge on Clinical Management and Outcomes in Patients Having a Curative Resection for Rectal Cancer. J Gastrointest Surg.21(12):2056-2065.

Appendix A

Meta-analysis studies

1. Ellis CT, et al. Evaluating Surveillance Patterns after Chemoradiation-Only Compared with Conventional Management for Older Patients with Rectal Cancer. J of the American College of Surgeons. 2019; 228(5):782-793. https://doi.org/10.1016/j.jamcollsurg.2019.01.010
2. Chapman W, et al. Total neoadjuvant therapy with short course radiation compared to concurrent chemoradiation in rectal cancer. Journal of Clinical Oncology. 2019; 37(4): 486-486. https://doi.org/10.1200/JCO.2019.37.4_suppl.486
3. Quezada-Diaz F, et al. Effect of Neoadjuvant Systemic Chemotherapy With or Without Chemoradiation on Bowel Function in Rectal Cancer Patients Treated With Total Mesorectal Excision. Journal of Gastrointestinal Surgery. 2019; 23(4):800-807. https://doi.org/10.1007/s11605-018-4003-7
4. Spiegel D, et al. Role of adjuvant chemotherapy following chemoradiation and surgery for locoregionally advanced rectal cancer: A Veterans Health Administration analysis. Journal of Clinical Oncology. 2018; 36(4):741-741. https://doi.org/10.1200/JCO.2018.36.4_suppl.741
5. Mancini R, et al. Tumor Regression Grade After Neoadjuvant Chemoradiation and Surgery for Low Rectal Cancer Evaluated by Multiple Correspondence Analysis: Ten Years as Minimum Follow-up. Clinical Colorectal Cancer. 2017;17(1):e13-19. http://dx.doi.org/10.1016/j.clcc.2017.06.004

6. Franke AJ, et al. Total Neoadjuvant Therapy: A Shifting Paradigm in Locally Advanced Rectal Cancer Management. Clinical Colorectal Cancer. 2017;17(1):1-12. http://dx.doi.org/10.1016/j.clcc.2017.06.008

7. Dossa F, et al. A watch-and-wait approach for locally advanced rectal cancer after a clinical complete response following neoadjuvant chemoradiation: a systematic review and meta-analysis. Lancet Gastroenterol Hepatol. 2017; 2(7): 501-513. http://dx.doi.org/10.1016/S2468-1253(17)30074-2

8. Kimberly P, et al. Complete Neoadjuvant Treatment for Rectal Cancer. American Journal of Clinical Oncology.2017; 40(3):283-287. https://doi.org/10.1097/COC.0000000000000149

9. Rodel C, et al. Rectal cancer: Neoadjuvant chemoradiotherapy. Best Practice & Research Clinical Gastroenterology. 2016; 30(4):629-639. http://dx.doi.org/10.1016/j.bpg.2016.06.004

Appendix B

NEWCASTLE - OTTAWA QUALITY ASSESSMENT SCALE

Note: A study can be awarded a maximum of one star for each numbered item within the Selection and Outcome categories. A maximum of two stars can be given for Comparability

Selection

1) Representativeness of the exposed cohort
   a) truly representative of the average _______________ (describe) in the community ✱
   b) somewhat representative of the average ______________ in the community ✱
   c) selected group of users eg nurses, volunteers
   d) no description of the derivation of the cohort

2) Selection of the non exposed cohort
   a) drawn from the same community as the exposed cohort ✱
   b) drawn from a different source
   c) no description of the derivation of the non exposed cohort

3) Ascertainment of exposure
   a) secure record (eg surgical records) ✱
   b) structured interview ✱
   c) written self report
   d) no description

4) Demonstration that outcome of interest was not present at start of study
   a) yes ✱
   b) no

Comparability

1) Comparability of cohorts on the basis of the design or analysis
   a) study controls for _____________ (select the most important factor) ✱
   b) study controls for any additional factor ✱ (This criteria could be modified to indicate specific control for a second important factor.)

Outcome

1) Assessment of outcome
   a) independent blind assessment ✱
   b) record linkage ✱
   c) self report
   d) no description

2) Was follow-up long enough for outcomes to occur
   a) yes (select an adequate follow up period for outcome of interest) ✱
   b) no

3) Adequacy of follow up of cohorts
   a) complete follow up - all subjects accounted for ✱
   b) subjects lost to follow up unlikely to introduce bias - small number lost - > ____ % (select an adequate %) follow up, or description provided of those lost) ✱
   c) follow up rate < ____% (select an adequate %) and no description of those lost
   d) no statement

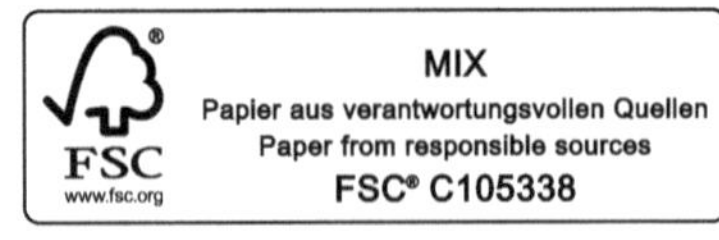

Printed by Books on Demand GmbH, Norderstedt / Germany